Endomorph Diet Reset

A 21-Day Meal Plan with Exercise to Activate Your Metabolism, Burn Fat, and Lose Weight by Eating More. Simple and Tasty Weight Loss and Health Improving Dishes

By

Mark R. Dickson

Disclaimer

Table of Contents

Introduction

Endomorph Diet is a new approach to weight loss and body transformation that focuses on the special requirements and problems that individuals who have an endomorph body type face in their quest to achieve their weight loss and body transformation goals. The Endomorph Diet is a diet that focuses on the specific requirements and hurdles that endomorph body types confront. The physique of endomorphs is typically more spherical and softer, and they have a slower metabolism. Additionally, endomorphs have a tendency to accumulate excess fat in their thighs and abdomen. There are a great number of endomorphs that exhibit these traits. Because of this, it may be extremely tough for individuals to reduce their body fat and meet the body composition objectives they have set for themselves.

The Endomorph Diet is a specialized eating plan that is designed to assist individuals with this body type in accomplishing their weight loss goals. This diet takes into account the specific challenges that endomorphs undergo and helps them overcome those challenges. It lays an emphasis on acquiring a balanced diet of macronutrients such as carbs, protein, and healthy fats, in addition to integrating foods that promote satiety, improve metabolism, and support general health. In addition, it incorporates meals that increase the likelihood of feeling full.

Endomorphs who are having problems losing weight and altering their body composition may find success with the Endomorph Diet, which offers a solution that is both sustainable and effective thanks to its evidence-based methodology and tailored recommendations. It is possible for you to accomplish your objectives and bring about great changes in your body with the help of the Endomorph Diet. A decrease in body fat, an increase in the amount of lean muscle mass you possess, or an improvement in your overall health could be among the changes that occur as a result of these practices.

Moreover,

Endomorphs have different nutritional and physical activity needs than other body types, such as ectomorphs and mesomorphs, according to the Endomorph Diet, which recognizes that not all body types are created equal and that the requirements of endomorphs are different from those of other body types. Endomorphs have a metabolic rate that is typically lower than that of other body types. This indicates that endomorphs burn fewer calories while they are at rest than other body types. Because of this, it might be more difficult for them to lose weight because they have to consume fewer calories than persons with other body types in order to attain the same level of calorie deficit.

The Endomorph Diet lays an emphasis not only on obtaining a balanced intake of macronutrients, but also on the value of ingesting nutrient-dense foods, such as fruits and vegetables, such fruits are abundant in a range of vitamins, minerals, and fiber. These meals not only serve to maintain overall health, but they also induce satiety and can assist endomorphs in feeling full and satisfied on a lower calorie intake.

The Endomorph Diet places a strong emphasis on physical activity, which studies have proven to be critical for both weight loss and overall health. Endomorphs may need to adjust their workout regimens to match their body type, focusing on activities that encourage fat-burning and muscle-building, such as high-intensity interval training (HIIT) and weightlifting. This will assist endomorphs in getting the most out of their workouts and reaching their fitness goals.

The Endomorph Diet, as a whole, presents a system that is both comprehensive and efficient for attaining weight loss and body transformation goals, and it does so by catering to the special requirements and problems experienced by persons who have an endomorphic body type. Endomorphs can reach their weight loss objectives and enhance their overall health and well-being by following the Endomorph Diet, which places a focus on eating a balanced diet, consuming foods that are rich in nutrients, and engaging in regular physical activity.

Chapter 1: What Exactly is an Endomorph

Endomorph is a term that is used to describe a specific body type that is prevalent in humans and is differentiated by a greater amount of overall body fat as well as a more rounded and gentler shape. persons who have endomorph body types often have metabolisms that are slower than those of persons with other body types, and they also have a propensity to accumulate weight more quickly. Additionally, they could be shorter than typical and have larger bones.

In the 1940s, an American psychologist by the name of William Sheldon suggested the idea that people may be categorized into three basic categories based on their physical qualities as well as the attributes that define their personalities. This was the origin of the concept that is today known as "body types." These three groupings were referred to as endomorphs, mesomorphs, and ectomorphs correspondingly.

People who are endomorphs are considered to have a "pear-shaped" figure because they tend to store more fat in the lower half of their bodies, notably in the buttocks, thighs, and hips. They might also have a larger face and a bigger waistline. It's crucial to highlight that not all endomorphs are necessarily obese or unhealthy, despite the fact that the term "endomorph" is usually used to refer to persons who are overweight. Individuals who fall within a healthy weight range can yet have endomorph body types. Endomorph body types can also be present in athletes.

The reason endomorphs often have larger levels of body fat is because their metabolism is normally slower than that of ectomorphs. Because of this, the rate at which their bodies burn calories is slowed, which makes it simpler for them to gain weight and more tough for them to shed weight. Endomorphs, on the other hand, may have a stronger inclination to store calories as fat, which, over time, can contribute to increasing levels of obesity and weight gain.

Endomorphs may have a more difficult time losing weight compared to persons with other body types; nonetheless, it is vital to bear in mind that weight loss is still feasible with a nutritious diet and constant physical activity. Endomorphs, on the other hand, might need to put in more effort and be more reliable in their food and exercise regimens in order to see any gains.

In terms of nutrition, endomorphs may benefit from a diet that is higher in protein and lower in carbohydrates, particularly processed carbohydrates like white bread and sugar. This can help to support weight loss by encouraging fullness and reducing cravings for meals that are high in calories but low in nutrients. Both of these things are excellent for weight loss.

Endomorphs should pay attention to both their diet and their activity levels on a constant basis. Even though any form of physical exercise has the potential to be beneficial, endomorphs, in particular, could do well to focus on activities that support the growth of muscle, such as weightlifting or resistance training. This can help to raise the individual's metabolic rate overall and encourage fat loss over the course of time.

Acquiring a grasp of bodily kinds
Accomplishing your fitness goals necessitates that you have a thorough awareness of the body type you possess. Every person has a specific body type, which influences not only their shape but also their metabolism and the other features of their physical makeup. Recognizing your body type allows you to tailor your exercise and nutrition routines to match your particular requirements, which, in turn, can lead to increased performance during your workouts and more satisfying overall results.

The following is a list of the three basic body types:

Ectomorphs have a thin, slender body with long limbs, small hips, and a rapid metabolism. Ectomorphs can be identified by their body type. They tend to have difficulties gaining weight and creating muscle and may need to consume more calories and engage in strength training to reach their desired physique.

Mesomorphs: Mesomorphs have a strong, athletic body with broad shoulders and small hips. They are more likely to be successful in sports that need strength and power, as they have a predisposition to acquire muscle and burn fat more easily. The combination of a good diet and consistent exercise is often highly beneficial for mesomorphs.

Endomorphs: Endomorphs have a rounder, broader build with wider hips and thicker bones.

They have a propensity to readily accumulate fat and may have a slower metabolism, all of which make it more difficult to eliminate excess pounds. Endomorphs may benefit from a lower-carbohydrate, higher-protein diet, and cardio and resistance training to assist in enhancing their metabolism.

People can have a combination of two or even three different body types, which is something that should be kept in mind. It is crucial to note that not everyone can be categorized neatly into one particular body type category.

You may establish what sort of body you have by utilizing a variety of methods, such as measuring the proportion of fat in your body, assessing the physical traits you possess, or obtaining the opinion of an expert in the field of fitness. As soon as you have an adequate grasp of your body type, you can start to change both your exercise regimen and your nutrition so that they better suit your demands.

Understanding your body type is vital to attaining your exercise goals and having a healthy lifestyle in general. You may maximize your outcomes and improve both your overall health and well-being if you take into account the individual characteristics of your body that are unique to you and alter your plan accordingly.

Endomorphic qualities in terms of their physical attributes

Endomorphs are people that have a body type that is defined by a larger and rounder frame, paired with a higher amount of body fat. Individuals with this body type seem to have a higher chance of having certain disorders. These people often have a slower metabolism, which makes it more tough for them to lose weight and sustain a leaner body over time. The following is a list of observable features that are usually connected with individuals who have an endomorph body type:

1. A soft, rounder body shape with a curvier appearance endomorphs often have a softer, rounder body shape than mesomorphs do. They have a propensity to be shorter and stockier in shape, with a larger waist and fuller hips than the normal person.

2. A high proportion of body fat Endomorphs often have a larger percentage of body fat compared to those with other body types, which might make it tougher for them to acquire a lean and toned appearance. This is owing to the fact that their bodies have a stronger inclination to retain fat, particularly in the abdominal region.

3. A slower metabolism Endomorphs, in comparison to those with other body types, have a metabolism that is slower, which indicates that they burn calories at a slower pace. Because of this, it may be more difficult for individuals to drop their weight and keep it at a healthy level.

4. Larger bones Endomorphs often have a larger bone structure than other body types, which is one element that contributes to their overall larger physique. This can be noted in their larger shoulders and hips, as well as their thicker wrists and ankles. Additionally, their hands and feet tend to be larger.

5. A more round face Endomorphs often have a more round face shape than mesomorphs, with larger cheeks and a more rounded jawline. They may look younger as a consequence of this, but it may be more difficult for them to obtain a chiseled and defined appearance as a result of this as well.

Endomorphs, in comparison to those with other body types, often have a softer, rounder appearance overall. In spite of the fact that this may make it more difficult for them to obtain a lean and toned body, it also bestows upon them a

one-of-a-kind appearance that may be charming
and desirable.

Chapter 2: Activate Your Body Metabolism

The term "metabolism" refers to all of the chemical reactions that take place in our bodies. These chemical reactions are responsible for keeping the organism alive and working properly. On the other hand, the word "metabolism" typically refers to the metabolic rate, commonly known as the number of calories that we burn. When our metabolic rate is higher, the number of calories that we burn and the ease with which we may lower our weight and keep it off are both boosted.

The quantity of calories that must be eaten by the body in order for it to function correctly while it is at rest, such as when we are sleeping or resting, is referred to as the basic metabolic rate. It is responsible for around 60–65 percent of the total energy expenditure. The core metabolic process does not take into consideration the number of calories necessary for all of the other activities that we engage in, such as moving our bodies (25-30%), thinking (5%-10%), and digesting meals (5%-10%). The number of calories burned during activities in addition to the number of calories burned while at rest make up our overall energy expenditure.

When people diet, their metabolism frequently slows down. The body puts up this kind of fight against the process of reducing weight. Although the reason for this phenomenon is a mystery, researchers believe that it is an old process. Because the first cells to form on Earth were unable to discover any nourishment, they were able to live by decreasing the quantity of energy they expended. This mechanism, which benefited mammals in surviving glacial eras and is still present in both animals and humans, was important to their survival.

How does one get their metabolism going?

When dieting, one of the problems is preventing one's metabolism from slowing down. Here are several methods that this barrier can, and the metabolism can be increased.

1. Eat more protein

Consuming food can offer our metabolism a momentary boost that lasts for a few hours. This process is known as trophic thermogenesis or the thermal effect of food, abbreviated TEF. It is related to the increased calories that are necessary for digestion, absorption, and digesting of meals. The breakdown of protein results in an increase in caloric expenditure. When compared to the effects of consuming carbs (5-10%) and fat (0-3%), the metabolic rate is enhanced by 15-30% when food thermogenesis occurs owing to the consumption of proteins.

Additionally, the more protein we ingest, the more probable it is that we will eat less calories overall. One study found that subjects had a tendency to consume about 440 fewer calories per day when the proportion of protein in their diet was increased from 15% to 30%, while the amount of carbohydrates they consumed remained the same, and there was a corresponding reduction in the amount of fat they consumed. According to what the researchers noted, the drop in calorie consumption may be linked to enhanced sensitivity in the central nervous system to leptin. Leptin is a hormone that is recognized to have a key function in lowering sensations of hunger.

2. Drink more water

People who use water instead of sugary beverages find it much simpler to manage their weight. Because it is a known truth that sugary drinks do contain calories, switching to water in favor of these beverages will invariably result in decreased calorie consumption. However, ingesting water can also momentarily speed up the body's metabolic processes.

The drinking of water can assist in the acceleration of metabolic rate, the elimination of waste from the body, and the regulation of hunger. In addition, drinking more water promotes your body to cease retaining water, which finally results in the elimination of those excess pounds of water weight that you have been lugging about. Dehydration, on the other hand, will induce a reduction in the rate at which your metabolism runs. In order to maintain sufficient hydration throughout the day, you should strive to take at least 10 to 12 glasses of water each day.

According to a number of studies, consuming around a half liter of water generates a 10%-30% increase in basal metabolic rate that lasts for approximately an hour. When drinking cold water, this effect on calorie burning can be exacerbated because the body must use more energy to get the water up to body temperature. Consuming water prior to meals may also result in a stronger feeling of fullness after eating.

3. Engage in severe physical activity and weight-lifting

The sort of exercise called high-intensity interval training comprises quick yet strong bursts of exertion. Even after exercise is ended, it can help the body burn extra fat by encouraging the metabolic rate to increase. According to the findings of a study conducted on young men who were overweight, this type of exercise over a period of 12 weeks reduced body fat by 2 pounds and belly fat by 17%.

Lifting weights is another wonderful technique to get your metabolism humming. This suggests that we burn more calories on a daily basis, even when doing nothing at all. Weight lifting helps preserve muscle mass and combats the decrease in metabolism that can occur when dieting alone results in weight loss. In one study, 48 overweight women adhered to a diet consisting of 800 calories per day, and some of them also participated in concurrent aerobic exercise or resistance training. Those who conducted workouts that emphasized resistance training were able to keep their muscular mass, metabolism, and strength. The others shrank in size, but during this time they also had a loss of muscle mass and a reduction in their metabolic rate.

4. Consume some coffee or oolong tea.

In certain trials, consuming green tea was found to improve metabolic rate by 4-5%, however, this was not the case in others. It achieves this by helping in the conversion of stored fat into free fatty acids, which in turn raises the amount of fat that is burned by 10-17%. There is evidence to show that drinking green tea while dieting helps speed up our metabolism.

The Maastricht University Medical Centre in the Netherlands did a review study that concluded that drinking green tea can boost your energy expenditure, generally known as the number of calories and fat grams that you burn each day. If you consume between one and three cups of green tea every day, you may notice that your body burns calories at a higher rate than it would have otherwise. In contrast to sugary juices, this is a lot better alternative to consider.

Additionally, coffee might speed up the metabolism by anywhere from 3 to 11%. It has comparable effects to green tea in that it helps the body burn fat. On the other hand, this tends to have a stronger influence on the more vulnerable ones. One study indicated that drinking coffee raised the amount of fat that was burned by 29% in lean women but only by 10% in obese women.

5. Nutrition

The majority of the foods you eat on a regular basis should be ones that help you burn fat and speed up your metabolism. Apples, dairy products (high in protein), salmon, eggs, lentils, avocado, red fruits (rich in antioxidants), pineapple, kiwi, lemon, ginger, cinnamon, grapefruit, and many other fruits and vegetables. Vegetables and Red fruits are usually high in antioxidants. Make sure that you are following a good fitness plan and that you are eating a balanced diet.

6. Sleep well

Are you aware that sleeping may not slow down or speed up the metabolism, but that not getting enough sleep can produce an imbalance and dysregulation of the hormones that control hunger and appetite? A lack of sleep can cause you to feel hungry, which can result in you nibbling in the middle of the night, experiencing a desire for sugar, and eventually consuming more calories than you should have. Because it slows down the metabolism, this energy surplus will eventually lead the person to gain weight.

Chapter 3: What is The Endomorph Diet

Some individuals feel that if you have an endomorph body type, it will be more difficult for you to lose weight than it will be for someone with a mesomorph body type to do the same thing.

There is really only one way to lose weight, and it does not matter what kind of body you have: you just have to make sure that you burn more calories than you take in. As long as you keep up this pattern, you will continue to reduce your body fat regardless of the meals that you consume in the meantime.

There is no such thing as a "perfect" diet that is going to work beautifully for everyone. We all have various requirements and schedules, therefore the greatest diet for you will be the one that you can stick to for the long haul.

An endomorph diet is one option. This type of diet places an emphasis on lean protein, healthy fats, and complex carbs while minimizing the intake of simple carbohydrates (white bread, added sugars, and processed foods). This diet shares aspects with the keto, Mediterranean, and paleo diets.

What exactly is involved in the endomorph diet?

Some individuals feel that if you have an endomorph body type, it will be more difficult for you to lose weight than it will be for someone with a mesomorph body type to do the same thing.

There is really only one way to lose weight, and it does not matter what kind of body you have: you just have to make sure that you burn more calories than you take in. As long as you keep up this pattern, you will continue to reduce your body fat regardless of the meals that you consume in the meantime.

There is no such thing as a "perfect" diet that is going to work beautifully for everyone. We all have various requirements and schedules, therefore the greatest diet for you will be the one that you can stick to for the long haul.

An endomorph diet is one option. This type of diet places an emphasis on lean protein, healthy fats, and complex carbs while minimizing the intake of simple carbohydrates (white bread, added sugars, and processed foods). This eating plan is comparable in many aspects to the ketogenic diet, the Mediterranean diet, and the paleo diet.

The dietary advice that is supplied by this plan is one that can be successfully followed not only by endomorphs but also by persons with other body types. It is in everyone's best advantage to have a diet that has a greater proportion of whole foods and a lower proportion of processed foods.

However, if your purpose is to use it as a tool for weight loss, it is crucial for you to keep your expectations in control and keep them reasonable. In most circumstances, it is a great deal more tough to keep the weight off than it was to get rid of the unwanted pounds in the first place. Rather than going on a crash diet for a short period of time, people who are successful at achieving a healthy weight often make changes to their lifestyle and make mindful selections about the foods they eat on a daily basis.

The endomorph diet is advantageous in many different ways.

The majority of the benefits that come from adhering to an endomorphic diet come from the weight loss that takes place as a direct result of doing so. There is an association between having an endomorph body type and having a higher prevalence of obesity. The United States is suffering from an epidemic of obesity, which affects more than forty percent of the adult population. Being obese or overweight boosts your chance of acquiring a variety of significant health disorders, including cardiovascular disease, diabetes, high blood pressure, and others.

Your health will improve if you can find a diet that not only helps you drop excess pounds but also allows you to keep them off. The endomorph diet, which focuses an emphasis on lean protein, healthy fats, and complex carbs, has several benefits, one of which is that it helps many people feel fuller with less food. Why? Because complex carbs, such as whole grains and veggies, are sources of energy that burn more slowly. Your blood sugar levels will rise, simple carbohydrates such as sweets and starchy foods will be digested quickly, and you will be encouraged to consume more calories than you require in order to maintain your present weight. The accumulation of fat can be induced by any and all of these factors.

Consuming foods high in heart-healthy fats like olive oil, avocados, and fatty fish like salmon may help you minimize your overall risk of developing heart disease, as well as lower your blood pressure and improve your cholesterol levels. Other examples of good fats include nuts, seeds, and avocados.

There are a few downsides to adopting the Endomorph Diet.
This eating plan can provide several obstacles that may be insurmountable for certain individuals, in addition to the paucity of large-scale, long-term studies on the endomorph diet and the body type diet as a whole.

The first difficulty to overcome is cutting down on the amount of carbohydrates consumed.

Your body probably produces an excessive quantity of insulin, which is likely the reason why it is unable to absorb carbs as efficiently as the bodies of others who have different body types. "I tell patients to eat more healthy fats." "I counsel patients to cut back on carbohydrates and increase their consumption of healthy fats."

Nuts, avocados, and olive oil are examples of foods that contain monounsaturated fats (MUFAs), which are also abbreviated as MUFAs.

The difficulty is that while it is simple to tell someone to consume less bread, rice, pasta, crackers, and potatoes, it is much more difficult to put this counsel into effect, particularly if you are accustomed to eating in this manner. This is especially true if you are trying to shed weight or enhance your health in some other way. As a consequence of this, keeping this kind of diet may be more challenging for certain people. For instance, one study found that persons with type 2 diabetes who followed a low-carb diet were able to lose weight and reduce the quantity of insulin they were taking when compared to those who did not follow such a diet. However, the researchers also discovered that it was unlikely for these individuals to continue following the diet after the initial period of six months had gone.

Another aim that may prove tough to attain is lowering the quantity of calories that one takes in each day. According to Catudal, an endomorph needs to have the most strict approach to their food. This contains the total calories as well as the quantity of calories that originate from carbohydrates. On the other side, an endomorph can experience weight loss if they do these activities. Even when you have reached your goals, you must keep the same routine of eating. If you do not, your body may revert to the state it was in when you initially started the program. The style of life that helped you reach this point is the way of life that you need to sustain if you want to stay in this place.

On the endomorph diet, you are allowed to consume the following categories of foods:

The endomorph diet plan places a larger emphasis on the consumption of foods that are high in complex carbs, healthy fats, and protein while limiting the consumption of foods that are high in simple carbohydrates. These sorts of foods are included:

Proteins: beef, chicken, turkey, eggs, salmon goods derived from milk and other dairy sources, such as yogurt, milk, and cottage cheese Fruits, in particular those that are low in carbohydrates, such as berries, melons, and avocados Fruits that are particularly low in carbohydrates include:

- Foods classed as vegetables, including high-fiber vegetables such as leafy greens, asparagus, and celery

In addition to being present in grains and starches, complex carbohydrates can also be found in starchy vegetables, legumes, and starchy vegetables like sweet potatoes and squash. Brown rice, quinoa, and other whole grains are examples of complex carbohydrates.

When it comes to **fats**, some examples of good fats include olive oil, avocados, almonds, and seeds.

On a diet tailored for endomorphs, you should avoid eating foods like these:

You should avoid consuming meals that are heavy in simple carbohydrates and sugar when you are following the endomorph diet, as well as the great majority of other diets, some examples of these foods are as follows:

- Candies, baked goods, pastries, and doughnuts are examples of foods that are high in sugar.
- Sweetened beverages like juices and soft drinks
- Simple carbs include meals like white bread and those that have additional sugars added to them (like some premade foods)

Exercises for endomorphs

If you want to successfully lose weight, your weight loss plan should incorporate some type of physical exercise such as cardio and strength training. This is true regardless of the type of physique you have. This technique is premised on the idea that participating in physical activity for longer periods of time leads to a greater loss of body fat through caloric expenditure.

HIIT, which stands for high-intensity interval training, is one sort of exercise that an endomorph (or anyone else) might think about performing. HIIT stands for high-intensity interval training. High-intensity interval training (HIIT) is an alternative to low-intensity steady-state cardio, often known as LISS. Instead of simply stepping on a treadmill and jogging for as long as you possibly can (also known as low-intensity steady-state cardio, or LISS), HIIT involves boosting your heart rate with intensive exercise such as sprinting, interspersed with lower-intensity recovery intervals of jogging or walking. During a typical high-intensity interval training (HIIT) session, you might sprint for one minute, then jog or walk for the next minute, and then sprint for the remaining 19 minutes of the session.

In addition to exercise, strength training, generally known as weight lifting, is essential for weight loss. It is possible that integrating weight training in your exercise program will result in an increase in your lean muscle mass and an improvement in your metabolic rate (the rate at which you burn calories), particularly when combined with cardio or aerobic exercise. You will boost your chances of effectively losing weight if you combine the various sorts of physical exercise outlined below with a reduction in the number of calories you consume each day.

Similar to dietary programs, there is no one exercise routine that is appropriate for everyone. Have a talk with your healthcare practitioner to ensure that the fitness objectives you establish and the routines you follow are acceptable for you. There is a vast selection of alternatives available, and you will want to choose one that is suitable for your body and that you will be able to adhere to over the long run.

Is the endomorph diet something that should be followed?

It doesn't matter what your body type is; if you choose a diet plan like the endomorph diet that promotes healthy eating and lower calorie consumption, you may discover that you lose weight more quickly. A diet that is too restricted, claims considerable weight loss in a very short length of time or tells you that you can skip exercising is a diet that should be avoided. The finest meal plan selections will be those that are sustainable over the long run.

Chapter 4: Macronutrients in The Endomorphs Diet

According to the somatotype theory, there is a type of diet known as the endomorph diet that is created for those who are naturally prone to carrying excess body fat. This type of individual is known as an endomorph. Endomorphs often have a metabolic rate that is slower than average, which can make it tough for them to shed weight and have a good body composition.

A larger proportion of protein and a lower proportion of carbs and fat are often included in the macronutrient ratios of an endomorph diet.

The following is a list of the suggested ratios of macronutrients for an endomorph diet:

1. Protein. It is recommended that endomorphs consume a larger proportion of protein in their diet, often anywhere between 35 and 40 percent of their total daily calorie intake. Lean cuts of meat, fish, eggs, and plant-based meals like beans, tofu, and tempeh are all excellent sources of protein. Other good options include poultry with a reduced fat level.

2. Carbohydrates. It is suggested that an endomorph ingest between 25 and 30 percent of their daily calorie intake from carbohydrates. Consuming complex carbs, such as whole grains, fruits, and vegetables, which include fiber and other nutrients that can help manage blood sugar levels, ought to be the main priority for everyone trying to lower their blood sugar levels.

3. Fat. It is recommended that endomorphs consume a modest quantity of fat, around thirty percent to thirty-five percent of their total daily calorie intake. On the other hand, it is vital to put an emphasis on the consumption of good fats, which may be found in foods such as nuts, seeds, avocados, and fatty fish.

Overall, the most important thing to keep in mind if you want your endomorph diet to be successful is to place an emphasis on eating nutrient-dense foods that promote weight loss and healthy body composition and to stay away from processed and high-calorie foods that can contribute to weight gain. In addition, you should make regular exercise and other forms of physical activity a part of your daily routine in order to support your attempts to reduce weight and enhance your overall health.

Chapter 5: Exercise For Endomorphs

Various somatotypes, which are another name for body types, respond favorably to a variety of physical activities. There are three unique body kinds, which are referred to as endomorphs, mesomorphs, and ectomorphs correspondingly. Each of these body types has its own unique traits. It's probable that the top workouts for endomorphs are going to look a little bit different than the top exercises for mesomorphs or ectomorphs.

"Endomorphs typically have a stockier build and store a lot of body fat," writes the author, who goes on to claim that endomorphs have a propensity to acquire weight relatively fast while simultaneously having difficulties shedding weight.

When it comes to the most effective forms of exercise for endomorphs, a combination of resistance training and cardiovascular work will produce the best results: "Endomorphs can increase their daily calorie expenditure by engaging in cardiovascular exercise, and resistance training can encourage the growth of muscle."

Endomorphs may wish to choose low-impact cardio activities such as incline walking or spinning depending on their body weight and the danger of damage. You can do incline walking on a treadmill, or you can choose a steep spot outside to do it in. Both options are good. Start with a minimum of 20 minutes of walking and progressively work up to longer sessions as your fitness improves.

"When it comes to strength training, you should consider working up to rep ranges of 12 to 15 for each exercise. This will not only help you build muscle, but it will also keep your heart rate higher on average during your workouts, which means that you will receive some benefit to your cardiovascular system from them as well.

Advice for endomorphs regarding their food, workout routines, and recuperation time
Long explains that when it comes to the topic of weight loss, endomorphs should focus first and foremost on their nutrition.

"In order for endomorphs to reduce body fat, they need to consider being in a calorie deficit, which implies that they are burning more calories than they are ingesting on a daily basis. They will be able to attain their weight loss objectives even if they do not make any alterations to their existing workout program if they increase their nutrition.

Endomorphs don't need to be concerned with their macronutrient breakdown (the proportion of calories they obtain from protein, carbohydrates, and fats), and instead should focus on maintaining a calorie deficit. Utilizing a calorie tracker such as My Fitness Pal is a great approach for keeping tabs on the number of calories you consume. This might provide beneficial insight into how much you may be consuming; usually, we consume a significant lot more energy than we feel we do.

Rest days should undoubtedly be incorporated into your fitness regimen; however, this does not mean that you should do nothing but lounge about all day. Walking and other forms of low-intensity aerobic exercise, such as swimming, are ideal strategies to continue physical activity during a rest day while still allowing the body to recoup.

The most efficient training programs for endomorphs

These are the most beneficial exercises that you should integrate into your regimen if you have an endomorph body type. Aim to complete two to four sets of each of the exercises indicated below, executing 12 to 15 repetitions in each set.

The bulk of these routines need the use of weights, and we've collected a list of the finest adjustable dumbbells for weightlifting at home for your convenience.

Squats

For this exercise, you can either use a barbell or grip a dumbbell on each shoulder.
Maintain your posture by standing up straight with your feet about shoulder-width apart and your toes turned out slightly. As you lower yourself into a squat position by pulling your hips back and bending your knees, try to keep your core engaged and your back flat. Get into a position where your thighs are at least parallel to the floor by lowering yourself. The next phase is to climb back up to a standing position by pushing up through the heels.

Squats with a resistance band may be done in a variety of ways, and we'll teach you how to execute each one below.

Deadlifts

Maintain a stance in which your feet are shoulder-width apart and the bar is positioned exactly above your feet, in front of your shins. Put your hips in a more rearward position, slightly bend your knees, and lean forward while maintaining a flat back and engaging your core. In addition, your neck ought to be in alignment with your back. Take hold of the bar and arrange your hands so that your palms are facing inward, right outside of your legs.

You should drive up to standing while bringing the bar up with you as you push through your feet. Maintain a straight arm stance, and once you're upright, give your glutes a firm squeeze. The next phase is to pull your feet together, bend your knees, and push your hips back as you carefully lower the bar to the floor while maintaining it close to your legs.

Lunges

You have various alternatives for how to perform this exercise: you can hold a barbell across your upper back, you can hold a dumbbell on each shoulder, or you can carry a single, heavier dumbbell with both hands, close to your chest. Maintain a straight stance with a level back and a forward look. Make a large stride forward with your left leg, bending at the knee and lowering yourself down as you do so. Your front right knee should be hovering just above the ground, and your front left toe should not be any more forward than your front knee. Your right knee should be raised slightly off the ground while you complete this exercise. Raise yourself back to the beginning posture by applying upward pressure via the front of the heel. After that, repeat the process with the opposite leg.

Learn how to perform lunges with the appropriate technique, as well as the benefits of doing them and the numerous versions you can try.

Pulldowns on the lats

The wider you make your grasp on the lat pulldown bar, the more work your lats are required to do while you complete the exercise. Maintain a straight back, plant both feet firmly on the ground, and hold the bar that is directly above you with your arms fully extended. After pausing, slowly raise the bar back up to the beginning position while continuing to pull it down to your upper chest area.

The following illustrates why lat pulldowns are such a great workout for training your back muscles:

Bench Press

Lie back on a flat bench with your feet flat on the floor and a barbell held straight over your shoulders. Check that the distance between your hands is slightly more than the width of your shoulders. This move may require the assistance of a spotter or a rack, especially if you are lifting a greater weight than usual.

Conceal your core muscles as you bring the bar down to your chest. After pausing, steadily press the bar back up to its initial position. During this exercise, you should keep your hips on the bench at all times, as arching your back increases the chance of injury and should be avoided at all costs.

Pressing the Shoulders
Holding a dumbbell by each shoulder with your palms facing forward, you should be standing erect (or you can do this exercise while sitting upright on a bench). It is recommended that the elbows be bent at a 90-degree angle.

As you extend your arms upward and press the dumbbells above your head, be careful to keep your back and core engaged. Next, bring the dumbbells back to the beginning position in a controlled manner.

Chapter 6: Best Endomorph Diet Supplements

Understanding the Endomorph Supplement Game

First things first, let's speak about why supplements matter for endomorphs. Your body has its distinct rhythm, and occasionally, it needs a little nudge to start things moving. That's where the correct supplements come into play. They aren't magic medicines, but they undoubtedly can be the allies you need in your quest for a healthier, more vibrant you.

Protein Powders: The Unsung Heroes

Meet the MVPs of the supplement world: protein powders. Endomorphs, rejoice! These powders are like the sidekicks you never knew you needed. Packed with muscle-loving goodness, they not only assist in muscle regeneration but also keep you feeling full, which is a superhero move in the war against overeating.

Usage Tip: Swap your typical snacks with a protein shake, and notice how your desires take a backseat.

Omega-3 Fatty Acids: The Brain and Body Protectors

Next up on our superhero list is omega-3 fatty acids. These bad boys are like shields for your brain and body. Endomorphs typically confront the issue of not simply dropping pounds but also ensuring their bodies function at their prime. Omega-3s accomplish just that, boosting heart health, and cognitive function, and even giving your metabolism a modest push.

Usage Tip: Consider adding fish oil supplements to your everyday regimen. Your heart and metabolism will appreciate you.

Vitamin D: The Sunshine Vitamin's Mighty Sidekick

Let's talk about the sunlight vitamin — Vitamin D. If you're an endomorph, you might not be getting enough of this golden delight. Vitamin D has a key role in weight management, and supplementing can be a game-changer. It's not just about strong bones; it's about a powerful metabolism too.

Usage Tip: Check with your healthcare professional about the correct Vitamin D supplement dosage for you. Sunlight in a pill — who knew?

Fiber Supplements: The Digestive BFFs

Fiber is the hidden hero of digestion. For endomorphs, keeping the digestive tract happy is vital, and fiber supplements can be your digestive BFFs. They keep things going smoothly, avoid overeating, and assist in that sensation of fullness that's frequently elusive.

Usage Tip: Introduce fiber supplements gradually to avoid any big surprises for your digestive system. Your belly will thank you later.

Caffeine: The Metabolism Booster with a Kick Who knew your morning cup of joe could be more than simply a wake-up call? Caffeine, the unsung hero in your coffee mug, is a metabolism stimulant. For endomorphs, it can be that extra push needed to rev up the engine and start burning calories.

Usage Tip: Enjoy your caffeine fix in moderation. It's about balance, not turning into a jittery Superman.

Endomorphs are persons who have a tendency to gain weight easily and a metabolism that is inherently slower than other people. They have a larger and more spherical body type, which makes it more difficult for them to shed weight and build muscle than it is for other people. They can, however, fulfill their fitness targets by following a suitable diet, engaging in the appropriate exercise program, and using the appropriate weight-loss supplements. This article will examine the finest weight supplements for endomorphs and how they can assist endomorphs in accomplishing their fitness objectives.

Protein derived from Whey.
Athletes, bodybuilders, and those who are just simply interested in becoming in better condition utilize whey protein as a weight gain supplement frequently. It is a complete protein, meaning that it contains all of the essential amino acids that are required for the maintenance and development of muscle tissue. Because it is simple to digest and the body can absorb it fast, it is an ideal choice for a supplement to take after exercise. Whey protein can assist endomorphs in building muscle mass and support weight loss by improving metabolism and reducing hunger. This helps endomorphs attain their exercise goals more successfully.

Creatine

Creatine is an amino acid that occurs naturally and can be found in the cells of your muscles. It contributes to the improvement of the generation of adenosine triphosphate (ATP), which is the cellular form of money for energy. Strength and performance can be improved by using creatine supplements in conjunction with high-intensity training. Additionally, it can assist endomorphs in increasing muscle mass and speeding up their metabolism, both of which make it simpler to lose weight.

Leucine, isoleucine, and valine are examples of essential amino acids that belong to the BCAA category of branched-chain amino acids, often known as BCAAs. Endomorphs can benefit from consuming BCAAs since they help them develop muscular mass, minimize muscle fatigue and soreness, and boost fat reduction. They also assist in avoiding the breakdown of muscle tissue, which can happen after very intense workouts or extended periods of calorie restriction.

Beta-Alanine

Endomorphs have the ability to boost their physical endurance and performance by taking beta-alanine, which is a non-essential amino acid. Increasing the quantities of carnosine in the muscle cells encourages them to operate, and this helps to buffer the buildup of lactic acid that occurs during high-intensity exercise. Endomorphs can benefit from using beta-alanine supplements since it enables them to power through their exercises and complete more reps, which in turn leads to improved muscle building and lower body fat.

Glutamine

Glutamine is the most frequent amino acid in the body and plays a crucial function in both the creation of proteins and the maintenance and repair of muscles. Additionally, it can help boost the immune system and minimize inflammation in the body. Supplementing with glutamine can assist endomorphs in recovering from their exercises more rapidly, lessen muscular pain and tiredness, and enhance their overall muscle mass. Additionally, it can help prevent the loss of muscle mass that might occur during periods of calorie restriction.

CLA

CLA, also known as conjugated linoleic acid, is a naturally occurring fatty acid that is capable of supporting endomorphs in lowering body fat while allowing them to preserve their muscular mass. It achieves this by lowering the activity of an enzyme in the body that is important for boosting the storage of fat. Taking a CLA supplement may also help improve insulin sensitivity, lower inflammation, and bring cholesterol levels down to healthier ranges.

Beta-hydroxy-beta-methylbutyrate, also known as HMB, is a metabolite of the amino acid leucine that has been found to assist endomorphs in increasing their muscle mass while simultaneously slowing their rate of muscle breakdown. It accomplishes this by raising the rate of protein synthesis in muscle cells while concurrently decreasing the rate at which protein is broken down. In addition to helping enhance endurance, taking an HMB supplement can also assist in lessening muscle discomfort.

In conclusion, endomorphs who desire to support their fitness goals by gaining weight may benefit from using weight supplements. The finest weight gain supplements for endomorphs include whey protein, creatine, BCAAs, beta-alanine, glutamine, CLA, and HMB. However, prior to introducing any nutritional supplements into your routine, it is vital that you explore your alternatives with a skilled medical practitioner or a licensed dietitian. A well-rounded diet, a consistent exercise routine, and proper rest are three of the most critical variables in obtaining and retaining a healthy weight as well as body composition.

Chapter 7: Endomorph Diet Plan

Sample Menu for an Endomorph Body Type Over the Course of 21 Days

The endomorph body type is characterized by a sluggish metabolism and a predisposition to gain weight rapidly. As such, individuals with an endomorph body type need to be careful about what they consume and how much they eat. A well-designed meal plan can help endomorphs maintain their weight and accomplish their health goals.

Here is a 21-day diet plan for endomorphs that contains nutrient-dense meals, moderate quantities, and a balanced macronutrient ratio.

Day 1
Breakfast: Greek yogurt, berries, almonds, and chia seeds
Mid-morning snack: Almond butter-covered apple slices

Lunch: Grilled chicken breast, mixed greens, avocado, and tomatoes.

Afternoon snack: Carrot and cucumber hummus.

Dinner: Grilled salmon with roasted veggies (broccoli, cauliflower, and carrots)

Day 2

Breakfast: Spinach, mushroom, and feta omelet.

Mid-morning snack: Peanut butter and banana.

Lunch: Whole-wheat turkey and Swiss cheese sandwich with fruit.

Afternoon snack: Greek yogurt with honey and nuts.

Dinner: Beef stir-fry with peppers, onions, zucchini, and brown rice.

Day 3

Breakfast: Almond milk-banana-cinnamon overnight oats

Mid-morning snack: Hard-boiled egg with celery sticks

Lunch: Grilled shrimp and quinoa salad.

Afternoon snack: Cottage cheese with pineapple chunks.

Dinner: Sweet potato and roasted Brussels sprouts with baked chicken breast

Day 4

Breakfast: Spinach, banana, berry, almond butter smoothie bowl.

Mid-morning snack: Nut and dried fruit trail mix

Lunch: Mixed greens, cucumber, and cherry tomato grilled chicken salad.

Afternoon snack: Sea salted edamame

Dinner: Beef and vegetable stew on whole-grain bread.

Day 5

Breakfast: Avocado toast and scrambled eggs.

Mid-morning snack: Cheese-covered apple slices

Lunch: Mixed greens, cherry tomatoes, and cucumber tuna salad.

Afternoon snack: Greek yogurt with granola and fruit.

Dinner: Grilled fish with roasted sweet potato and green beans

Day 6
Breakfast: Banana, nut, and maple syrup quinoa bowl.
Mid-morning snack: Hummus-covered baby carrots

Lunch: Grilled chicken wrap with mixed greens, avocado, and tomatoes
Snack: Mixed berries with whipped cream.
Dinner: Brown rice and beef-broccoli stir-fry

Day 7
Breakfast: Greek yogurt parfait with granola, berries, and honey.
Mid-morning snack: Banana with almond butter
Lunch: Whole-wheat turkey and Swiss cheese sandwich with fruit.
Afternoon snack: Cottage cheese with chopped peaches.
Dinner: Grilled chicken breast with roasted sweet potato and asparagus.

Day 8

Breakfast: Spinach scrambled eggs and whole-grain bread.

Mid-morning snack: Nut and dried fruit trail mix

Lunch: Mixed greens, cucumber, and cherry tomatoes with grilled shrimp.

Afternoon snack: Greek yogurt with honey and nuts.

Dinner: Baked salmon, quinoa, and roasted veggies (bell peppers, onions, and zucchini)

Day 9

Breakfast: Spinach, banana, berry, almond butter smoothie bowl.

Snack: Hummus-covered baby carrots

Lunch: Grilled chicken wrap with mixed greens,

Day 10

Breakfast: Banana-nut oatmeal with honey.

Mid-morning snack: Almond butter-covered apple slices

Lunch: Grilled chicken breast, mixed greens, avocado, and tomatoes.

Afternoon snack: Cottage cheese with pineapple chunks.

Dinner: Roasted Brussels sprouts, sweet potato, and baked salmon.

Day 11

Breakfast: Greek yogurt, berries, almonds, and chia seeds

Mid-morning snack: Nut and dried fruit trail mix

Lunch: Whole-wheat turkey and Swiss cheese sandwich with fruit.

Afternoon snack: Sea salted edamame

Dinner: Beef stir-fry with peppers, onions, zucchini, and brown rice.

Day 12

Breakfast: Avocado toast and scrambled eggs.

Mid-morning snack: Hummus-covered baby carrots

Lunch: Mixed greens, cucumber, and cherry tomatoes with grilled shrimp.

Afternoon snack: Greek yogurt with granola and fruit.

Chicken breast on the grill, sweet potatoes, and green beans to roast for supper.

Day 13

Breakfast: Spinach, banana, berry, almond butter smoothie bowl.

Mid-morning snack: Cheese-covered apple slices

Lunch: Mixed greens, cherry tomatoes, and cucumber tuna salad.

Afternoon snack: Cottage cheese with chopped peaches.

Dinner: Sweet potato and roasted Brussels sprouts with baked chicken breast

Day 14

Breakfast: Banana, nut, and maple syrup quinoa bowl.

Mid-morning snack: Nut and dried fruit trail mix

Lunch: Grilled chicken wrap with mixed greens, avocado, and tomatoes

Snack: Berries with whipped cream.

Dinner: Brown rice and beef-broccoli stir-fry

Day 15

Breakfast: Greek yogurt parfait with granola, berries, and honey

Mid-morning snack: Banana with almond butter

Lunch: Turkey and Swiss cheese sandwich on whole wheat bread with a side of fruit

Afternoon snack: Hummus with carrots and cucumber

Dinner: Grilled fish with roasted sweet potato and asparagus

Day 16

Breakfast consisted of eggs cooked with spinach and bread made with nutritious grains.

Mid-morning snack: Trail mix with almonds and dried fruit

Lunch: Grilled shrimp salad with mixed greens, cucumber, and cherry tomatoes

Afternoon snack: Greek yogurt with honey and nuts

Dinner: Baked salmon with quinoa and roasted vegetables (bell peppers, onions, and zucchini)

Day 17

Breakfast: Omelet with spinach, mushrooms, and feta cheese

Mid-morning snack: Baby carrots with hummus

Lunch: Grilled chicken breast with a mixed greens salad, avocado, and tomatoes

Afternoon snack: Cottage cheese with pineapple chunks

Dinner: Beef stir-fry with mixed vegetables (peppers, onions, and zucchini) with brown rice

Day 18

Breakfast: Overnight oats with almond milk, banana, and cinnamon

Mid-morning snack: Apple slices with almond butter

Lunch: Turkey and Swiss cheese sandwich on whole wheat bread with a side of fruit

Afternoon snack: Edamame with sea salt

Dinner: Sweet potato and roasted Brussels sprouts with baked chicken breast

Day 19

Breakfast: Smoothie bowl with spinach, banana, berries, and almond butter

Mid-morning snack: Trail mix with almonds and dried fruit

Lunch: Grilled chicken wrap with mixed greens, avocado, and tomatoes

Day 20

Breakfast: Greek yogurt with granola, berries, and honey

Snack for mid-morning: banana with almond butter

Lunch: Tuna salad with mixed greens, cherry tomatoes, and cucumber

Cottage cheese with chopped peaches as an afternoon snack

Dinner: grilled chicken with roasted sweet potato and green beans

Day 21

Breakfast: Scrambled eggs with whole-grain bread and sliced avocado

Mid-morning snack: Baby carrots with hummus

Lunch: Grilled shrimp salad with mixed greens, cucumber, and cherry tomatoes

Afternoon snack: Mixed berries with a dab of whipped cream

Dinner: Beef and broccoli stir-fry with brown rice

Endomorphs tend to have a slower metabolism, which makes it vital for them to focus on nutrient-dense foods that are high in protein, healthy fats, and complex carbs to maintain a healthy weight. This 21-day diet plan for endomorphs focuses on a combination of lean protein, complex carbohydrates, and healthy fats. It includes plenty of fresh fruits and vegetables to provide a range of vitamins and minerals, and it also gives healthy snack options to keep hunger at bay between meals. However, it's important to note that individual needs and preferences may differ, so it's always better to consult a trained dietician or healthcare expert before making any significant changes to your diet.

Chapter 8: Maintaining a Healthy Weight For Life

The Method That Is Proven to Be the Most Successful When It Comes to Long-Term Weight Loss

Is diet more important? Or exercise? Or neither?

Is diet more important? Or exercise? Or neither? In this section, we go into the study and debate the topic with a nutritionist in order to learn how to lose weight and maintain the loss over the long term.

There are a number of various methods to assess if someone is healthy, and their weight is just one of them. Having said that, lowering one's body mass is a typical desire for many persons who are seeking to enhance their health. There are a variety of advantages that come with reducing a few pounds by healthy means, such as greater control of blood sugar levels, lower risk of developing chronic diseases, and healthier blood pressure. And despite the fact that you have most likely been advised that appropriate eating and physical activity might lead to weight loss, the reality is that it is far simpler to say than to accomplish.

The route to a healthy weight and the ability to keep it off are both impacted by your general way of life. Diet and exercise work hand in hand; you can't rely on just one of them to bring you to your health and fitness goals. However, at different moments in your journey to reduce weight, they may be more useful to you than others. The question therefore is, what is the most effective approach for losing weight and keeping it off?

How is it that losing weight is different from retaining the same weight?
Although "calories in, calories out" is a frequent conceptual model for weight loss, it's not nearly as basic as that. There are a lot of various elements that might determine how many

calories you need to consume each day, such as your age, activity level, body composition, illness, injury, and more. Our metabolism can also be thought of as the amount of energy, or calories, that are consumed by our bodies on a daily basis.

There are three ways in which our bodies might burn calories, in addition to the calories that we burn when we exercise:

- Metabolic rate at rest (how much energy is needed to maintain your heart pumping and lungs breathing)Impact of food on body temperature (the energy it takes to digest what we consume)
- Thermogenesis from activities other than exercise (think of walking to work or going up the stairs).
- Our basal metabolic rate utilizes the great majority of the energy that is available in our bodies.

The process of reducing weight can actually have the effect of slowing down our metabolism (think: a smaller body uses less energy to heat than a larger one). That in and of itself isn't necessarily a negative thing, but it does indicate that in order to be effective in your efforts to reduce weight, you'll need to utilize a little bit more planning. Let's break down your primary emphasis for weight reduction versus maintaining your weight, as well as the distinctions between the two.

The Single Most Important Aspect of Successful Weight Loss
Establishing a calorie deficit, often known as eating fewer calories than your body burns in a day, is one of the most prevalent ways for weight loss. There are various ways to lose weight, but one of the most prevalent techniques is consuming fewer calories than your body uses in a day. "According to the findings of multiple research, exercise is not the key to successful weight loss. It is vital to have a calorie deficit in order to lose weight, and studies have shown

that it is simpler to develop and sustain a calorie deficit through dietary adjustments than it is through physical exercise "advises Younkin.

Therefore, while you are initially getting started, it is advisable to concentrate on the duties at hand rather than going to the gym on a daily basis. You are in luck because we offer a choice of meal plans for weight loss that can accommodate anyone's preferences.

However, embarking on a diet that significantly limits your food intake will not result in long-term weight loss. "Going on a diet is not the way to reduce weight in a healthy and permanent way. Younkin proposes that rather than significantly cutting calorie consumption in order to lose a considerable amount of weight in a short period of time, dieters should try to develop a tiny calorie deficit that they are able to maintain over time. "This can be accomplished by eating smaller portions, increasing one's consumption of vegetables and proteins, and decreasing one's consumption of simple carbohydrates, sugar, and alcohol,"

The Single Most Important Aspect of Keeping the Same Weight "After you've lost five to ten percent of your body weight, doctors recommend staying at that weight for at least six months before attempting to lose weight again (that is if you still have weight to lose). Your set point is the weight range that your body likes to stay in." Despite this, it is widely recognized how tough it is to keep off weight. According to the findings of a study that was published in BioPsychoSocial Medicine, approximately seventy percent of people were unable to maintain a ten percent weight decrease over the course of two years. Despite the fact that this may create the sense that the odds are stacked against you, it is feasible to successfully maintain one's weight by redirecting one's attention away from habits connected with weight loss.

When it comes to getting off weight and keeping it off for good, research reveals that exercise may be more essential than nutrition. Daily exercise that spans from moderate to high intensity is the single most important feature that connects persons who have successfully lost weight and kept it off. According to the findings of a study that was published in the journal Obesity, those who successfully dropped an average of 58 pounds and managed to keep it off exercise for roughly 40 minutes every day. This workout didn't have to be done all at once; rather, it could be split up into 10-minute portions and spread out throughout the day.

But if modifying your diet was the key to your weight loss in the first place, why is exercise deemed more important? The calorie count is the most crucial aspect to consider. A calorie deficit is important for weight loss, but maintaining a healthy weight demands a calorie balance, which implies there should be neither a shortfall nor an excess of calories.

People who exercised regularly were able to burn more calories during the day, which in turn allowed them to consume more food without feeling a calorie surplus.

"If you can't sustain a certain way of eating for the rest of your life, then you won't see the effects for the rest of your life. Therefore, in order to keep the weight off, any alterations you make to your diet need to be maintained if you want to keep the weight off, suggests Younkin. This explains why people who follow diets that are too restrictive tend to gain back the weight they lost (and then some). It's just not possible to keep up with those rigorous dietary requirements.

Suggestions for Preserving a Healthy Body Weight "Most of the time, people set unrealistic weight loss objectives. "If you're constantly thinking about food and your body in order to keep a certain number on the scale, that's not the healthiest weight for you," Younkin adds. "If you are restricting your food intake, over-exercising, or constantly thinking about food and your body in order to maintain a certain number on the scale, then you are not at your healthiest weight." It is vital that any changes you make in order to reduce weight be ones you can stick with in the long run. We are fortunate in that minor changes made with enthusiasm can result in considerable development over time.

The following tips are for persons who are striving to eat in a way that is consistent with their objectives of losing weight: "Aim to eat every three to four hours to maintain blood sugar balanced, schedule nutritious snacks, and don't feel guilty when you eat something you feel like you shouldn't.

People make it their goal to adhere to the healthy plate strategy around 80% of the time throughout the week and to not stress out about the remaining 20%. According to the healthy plate method, you should fill half of your plate with vegetables, a quarter of your plate with whole grains, and the remaining quarter of your plate with lean protein. With this strategy, limiting portion size is straightforward and does not involve painstaking measurements of everything. In addition, Younkin observes that "Being conscious of sugar and alcohol intake can also help," explaining that this is because "empty" calories have the ability to mount up over time.

Find a form of physical activity that you find pleasure in so that you won't dislike working out. Maintaining coherence will be simplified as a result of this. "However, when it comes to exercising, you should begin carefully and not go all out. Younkin gives the optimistic words, "Something is better than nothing." Walk for 10 or even twenty minutes if you only have half an hour available for a rigorous workout; save the other half of the hour for a more extensive session at a later time. If you feel like you've reached a plateau or are caught in a rut, try mixing up what you're doing or attempting something altogether new.

Lastly, accountability is a great tool that can assist you in maintaining the adjustments to your healthy lifestyle. Younkin says that if you don't want to have to do everything by yourself, you seek some aid from a buddy, hire a dietician, or cooperate with a personal trainer.

Conclusion

As we close up our 21 days together, it's not the end—it's a springboard for your continued adventure. Think of it as graduating from the 21-day crash course, not waving farewell to a routine. We've sparked a spark, and now it's time to convert it into a roaring fire.

You've tackled the obstacles, cherished the successes, and ideally, discovered a new enthusiasm for life. Maybe you found joy in the kitchen, experimenting with recipes you never thought you'd attempt. Perhaps those regular exercises became a routine, a moment you value for yourself.

But, well, this is just the beginning. It's like we've handed you the keys to a sleek new car; now, it's your turn to take it for a drive. Beyond these 21 days, there's a whole highway waiting for you—a highway of unlimited possibilities.

Remember, this isn't about reaching a finish line; it's about embracing a lifestyle that makes you feel wonderful. So, as you go into the world post-21 days, think of it as a big adventure. Sure, there can be detours and speed bumps, but those are just part of the beautiful route.

You've learned to relish nutrient-packed meals and discovered the joy of moving your body. Carry that wisdom with you, not as a rulebook but as a compass. Your path is uniquely yours, and the 21-day plan was only the compass needle pointing you in the proper direction.

Let's not call it a conclusion. No, let's call it a beginning. Commencement of a better, happier you. You're not stepping off the train; you're moving tracks to an express line of vitality. The 21 days were a sneak peek into the possibilities, and now it's time to create your narrative.

Here's to more tasty meals, exciting workouts, and a life that's not just about counting days but making each day count. So, keep that spark burning, and let the voyage continue. Your narrative doesn't end here; it unfolds brilliantly with every choice you make.